Dealing with Disability

DEALING

– with –

DISABILITY

Moving towards acceptance,
transformation
& renewal

Victoria Cairns

Matador
9 Priory Business Park,
Wistow Road, Kibworth Beauchamp,
Leicestershire, LE8 0RX
Tel: 0116 279 2299
Email: books@troubador.co.uk
Web: www.troubador.co.uk/matador
Twitter: @matadorbooks

ISBN 978 1789017 779

British Library Cataloguing in Publication Data.
A catalogue record for this book is available from the British Library.

Printed and bound in Great Britain by 4edge Limited
Typeset in 12pt Bembo by Troubador Publishing Ltd, Leicester, UK

Matador is an imprint of Troubador Publishing Ltd

CONTENTS

PART IV *Postscript*

Appendix

PART I

MY STORY

CHAPTER ONE

Introduction

OCTOBER 20TH 2017. Last night I dreamt I was standing and that I took three little steps shuffling forwards. That told me that my brain has not forgotten that I used to walk, and that I hope that I may be able to manoeuvre myself about moderately well using my arms somehow one day in the future.

Apparently I was told several times in my first months in hospital that I may never walk again, but I do not remember as I was probably too ill to hear and comprehend what people were saying. Later a physiotherapist told me that I should not assume that I would be able to walk again, but that I should remain optimistic. This was followed by: "You can have a good life in a wheelchair." Of course I cried, but, despite the first shock, this encouraged me, particularly when I thought of my two relatives in wheelchairs who have good lives and do enjoy themselves. My husband said that I can continue to do many of the things I have always enjoyed, such as chatting with friends, reading and watching films.

I was encouraged by the book *The Healing Power of Mind* by Tulku Thondup, which contains ideas in common with recent discoveries in neurology about brain regrowth and healing. This overlap with Eastern traditions is recognised in the preface of the book, *The Brain's Way of Healing*, by Norman Doidge. It inspired me to fight on, and I realised that to some extent much will depend on my attitude and how hard I work on exercises to rebuild certain abilities.

Certainly it is a struggle, and inevitably I have sometimes felt downhearted. One time when I was in a lot of pain that never seemed to stop, a nurse in the neurology ward said very gently, "Don't cry, it makes me sad if you cry." And another time, when I was with an occupational therapist, I said, "I am having a bad day," and then sobbed, "I hate being a cripple." I will never forget her comforting me and giving me a hug. I could often hear the nurses near me in the neurology ward talking to very distressed patients: "Don't worry, sweetheart, I am here next to you, and you are quite safe." The comfort that so many of us have received is never forgotten.

My cousin Eva has said to me that I should say "Thank you". Being a nurse, she knows what it means to the recipient. I had assumed it was obvious that I was grateful for any help, but I now see that it is important to show how much you appreciate what others are doing for you. They will feel better to know they are acknowledged and valued.

It may be hard for others to imagine that when we are so very vulnerable and weak as patients, the comfort that is given makes such a difference. Encouragement also is a huge help, as it so easy to become low and discouraged. This is a time to develop some inner strength, and it does help to have support.

CHAPTER TWO

The cause of my spinal cord injury

I N 2016 I suffered from increasingly disturbing episodes of a disorder known as atrial fibrillation, which is a form of irregular heart rhythm. As mentioned in Chapter 15, it is possible that my atrial fibrillation was a long-term result of having had Lyme disease, a bacterial infection caught from a tick. Atrial fibrillation can lead to a blood clot forming inside the chambers of the heart, which may result in having a stroke. I was therefore taking the drug apixaban, a blood-thinner to prevent a blood clot forming, but it led to my having some troublesome side-effects, including dizziness and weakness. It was becoming a burden, and I was often woken in the night by feeling my heart beating strangely. At the time, a friend said she had noticed that I was really not looking well. I bought a heart monitor so that I could record what was happening. In December, after two episodes, each lasting more than 12 hours and leaving me feeling very weak, I decided to go ahead with having an operation to solve the problem. I did not want to continue with the medication and thought an operation was the preferred alternative. The procedure, which is called ablation, involves inserting a thin, flexible wire called a catheter into the heart, and then using heat or cold to destroy the area of the heart muscle that is triggering the arrhythmias. I knew that this keyhole surgery carried a slight risk and that ablation can sometimes cause a little bleeding where the catheter was inserted.

In January 2017, I had the operation to deal with the area of my heart that was causing the abnormal heart rhythms. Unfortunately it resulted in a perforation of my heart. This is a known potential complication that occurs in about 1 percent of cases, around half of which then require heart surgery. The perforation led to significant bleeding around my heart which compressed it and stopped it from beating properly. The cardiologist inserted an emergency tube into the space around my heart to drain the blood but then, unfortunately, the blood at the back of the heart clotted and this pressed on the veins draining from my lungs into the heart, which resulted in a cardiac arrest. It was my bad luck that the only nearby operating theatres were occupied by two emergency patients, so I required a prolonged resuscitation for 90 minutes before I could have the open-heart surgery that I needed to remove the blood clot and fix the bleeding area. The prolonged resuscitation led to reduced output of blood from my heart and low blood pressure, which resulted in damage to my spinal cord and, to a lesser extent, to my brain. I also had a series of brain seizures, probably because my body was receiving such a shock. This has left me with a spinal cord injury, known as T8 incomplete, and slight brain damage. I am unable to walk or move my legs normally, and I have some difficulties focusing on images, thinking mathematically and remembering things. Such prolonged resuscitation often results in severe brain damage, or even death. My survival and minimal brain injury are a tribute to the skill of the resuscitation team.

I remained in a coma for nine days and in intensive care for a month. My husband, parents, brothers and Eva came to see me while I was in intensive care. Despite not actually remembering it, I have recently had the feeling that a wave of comfort ran through me whenever one of them said they were there right next to me. Around that time Eva told her mother that she should come and sing to me a song from my childhood, so she came and sang "Waltzing Matilda".

I started to join in by mouthing the words, and this was the first sign that I could hear and understand what was going on around me. Until then I had only occasionally and very briefly opened one eye. Music and of course talk can be very helpful for patients in a semi-conscious state.

I then spent over three months in the John Radcliffe Hospital in Oxford and four months in the Oxford Centre for Enablement. So altogether I spent nearly eight months in hospital, but was then able to come home in August.

In the month before I came home my husband had our house converted to be wheelchair-friendly. Luckily our house has one main floor downstairs, and it is small and suitable for conversion. The dining-room was changed into my bedroom and the nearby utility room was converted into a shower and bathroom with wheelchair access. The floor of the new bedroom was lifted to be at the level of the living room, and two doors were widened so that I can wheel myself about on the ground floor. I cannot go up to the bedroom upstairs, but a ramp was built next to the living-room so that I can wheel myself outside. We also now have a video door entry kit so that I can see who is outside the front door, speak to them and press a button to let them in.

I was very worried at first about coming home as I still need a lot of help throughout the day. After so many months of continuous care, with nurses ready to come whenever I pressed the bell, I was very anxious about how my husband and I could cope. My husband had to call 30 different agencies before he could find one that agreed to provide some care for me at home. We now have carers coming in twice every day, and that is working very well. I also see a physiotherapist regularly.

Unfortunately, there is a limited amount of home care available, and long-term home care is often only provided by the British National Health Service (NHS) if the patient clearly has no ability to cover any of the costs. The NHS also no longer provides regular physiotherapy after the patient has left hospital and is at home, although continuing physiotherapy is very important (see Chapter 12). It is possible to contact an organisation for support or advice, such as the Spinal Injury Association, or Age UK. Another is Care UK, which works closely with the NHS and provides advice to family carers who often feel overwhelmed. Details on these organisations are given at the end of this book.

PART II

MENTAL ATTITUDE

CHAPTER THREE

Brain recovery

A FTER I BECAME a good bit better, I realised that my brain had been fuzzy much of the time I was in hospital, and also that I was very distracted by spending so much energy and mental effort focusing on dealing with physical issues, and by the steady discomfort and pain I had throughout the day, I was therefore not very aware of what was going on around me and did not listen carefully to other people.

Over the months I was in hospital, I began to return very gradually to my old self. Oddly, I have had a lot of flashbacks of different memories from my childhood, as if a part of my brain was having a sleep while the rest was busy reactivating old thoughts. Old memories have been surfacing at least once a day over the past year, so there have been hundreds of them. I am surprised that there are so many memories stored there that until now I have often not been aware of.

It is a bit like reliving some of my life. Having the recurring childhood memories somehow fits with my husband saying that I regressed for a while and became rather childish. I am glad to say that I am now a bit more mature and my brain is slowly recovering. I have also had flashbacks of many of my later years as well.

When we were young, my two brothers and I often read books about pioneers roaming the American midwest, and we watched TV films like *Rawhide*, *Bonanza* and *Star Trek* (with Captain Kirk ready "to boldly go where no man has gone before"), and *Superman* (who "fights a never-ending battle for truth, justice, and the American way"). Nearly 50 years later those memories are still firmly embedded in my brain, and I can still sing the songs and recite the opening lines of some of those films. It shows how the books that children read and the films that they see can have a long-lasting effect, and the impressions remain.

I have forgotten how to do a few things like editing and storing Word files on the computer, but am gradually relearning what I need to. I have some damage on the right side of my brain, and I have a definite deterioration in my mathematical abilities and with how I process images. I have an inattention disorder and I do not pay attention to what I see on my left side. So the right side of my brain is dormant and idle, but I hope it is gradually recovering. Meanwhile it seems as if the left side of my brain, which is the more verbal side, is alive and active, possibly because it is freer to take over. Therefore I am writing this book. I am still able to speak German as before, but my spelling of English and German is unreliable. I know how the words sound, but what I have written often looks odd to me and has errors. I have a similar problem with recognising faces and instead listen to people's voices or think of facts about how they look, like their hair colour. When I feel that it is time, I will add some right-brain exercises to the long list of exercises that I do.

I have already started to help my 13-year-old god-daughter with her school maths. It is rather embarrassing that I have struggled with it a bit, but it is good for me, and I am now slowly returning to normal. I remember that I enjoyed algebra at that age, and now that I have to relearn things, it is like being at school again.

I feel very inspired by the book *The Brain That Changes Itself* by Norman Doidge, which I read some years ago. It is about the amazing ability of parts of the brain to regrow when needed, known as plasticity. The brain can reorganise itself and form new neural connections, and this can happen throughout life. The neurons (nerve cells) in the brain can compensate for injury and disease and adjust their activities in response to new situations or to changes in their environment. That has made me confident that my brain will return more or less to what it was, and I can already see I have improved mentally a lot over the months.

For most of 2017 my brain often thought I saw flashing white lights coming up on my left side. Those flashing lights have now mostly stopped, which indicates again that some brain recovery has taken place.

I have faith in the human body's general ability to recover and fix itself. I had a tube down my nose and throat giving me water and nourishment for nearly three months, which has left me with a rather hoarse voice. I used to sing soprano in a choir but I now cannot sing any high notes. In the first few weeks after the tube was removed I could only whisper and I coughed a lot. Gradually my voice has become stronger, and I believe that my body will sort the problem out by itself. The voice therapist in the hospital said that I may not be able to sing again, but I hope for the best and am very patient, even if it takes another year or two from now. Singing used to be one of my favourite activities. Highlights for me in recent years were summer singing holidays with our choir in

France and Spain, taking part in a singing course at the Verrochio Art Centre in Tuscany, and singing in a group as part of the Oxford Lieder Festival.

I have told the conductor of our choir that I will sing tenor one day if necessary. If I have to learn how to sing low notes after having always sung the tune along the top as a soprano, then I will work on training my brain to do that. I can manage some deep voices (although not particularly well), and so I occasionally sang along with Elvis Presley while on the standing frame in the physiotherapy gym. That cheered me up.

For most of 2017, whenever I took a deep breath I felt a pain like a bruise all across the front of my lungs, and I was very careful not to sneeze or cough too violently. This may have been because I had a few cracked ribs from having had my chest banged repeatedly when my heart stopped beating during the operation, or because the front of my chest was cut open to get access to my heart during the operation. After almost a year, the natural healing has taken place and the pain has nearly faded away.

Also, one by one, the various infections and skin problems I had in 2017 have been fixed. Clearly, the body can do a lot of natural healing by itself.

CHAPTER FOUR

Perseverance

REMEMBER WHEN I was nearly three years old my grandfather squatted down to look right into my eyes and give me an intense look which I understood and remembered it meaning: "Be strong in your life." I knew he was Daddy's Daddy, so for me he was a powerful person. We were going to live in Africa and he knew he would never see me again as he was ill with cancer. He was a neurosurgeon in Oxford, and they say he was very strong and determined, and believed very much in his patients being encouraged to work hard.

While I was in hospital, I would sometimes lie in bed at night and imagine him hovering above me. I am sure that if he were still alive today he would say: "Come on, keep going, work hard, and don't give up." I therefore must not give up.

There was a young patient near me in hospital, and when I was finally leaving to go home, I went to his room to say goodbye and said, "Be strong." He replied that he would. He was recovering very slowly after a serious accident, and I do hope that he has remained mentally strong. That would be my advice to all patients in a similar situation: you have to hang on and persevere, even though it is tough.

CHAPTER FIVE

Avoiding negative thoughts

THINK IT is important in life not to dwell too long on negative thoughts. The person that suffers from those thoughts is you. I was told in hospital that I should try not to think too much in black and white, and so not about either I will walk again or I will never walk again. That was a good suggestion which did help me to try to dwell less on it, as I had been, with my thoughts going back and forth over the open question. I was also told that I should think about the things I can do and not think about what I cannot do. I immediately thought about helping my godchildren with their school maths. That is something I have done for years and will continue to do, and I can do it without being able to walk. That thought made me feel more valuable and less of a burden. There are many things one can do on the phone or on a computer, even when in a wheelchair.

For many months after my operation a wave of distress would hit me every ten days or so. It was as if the thoughts were hovering constantly in the back of my mind and they would suddenly be triggered and would surge forward. It felt like a chemical force in my brain that I could not stop. But I did think each time that I would feel different the next day, and it is true that I did. I am pleased to say that the recurrent surges of negative feelings have now stopped and I no longer get the waves of despair.

It can seem hard at first to avoid the negative thoughts, but it is possible to break the pattern. It is known that excessive empathy and sharing the negative emotions of others may result in an increase in negative feelings, and it may lead to eventual burn-out, so it is best to avoid that if possible. Being over-sympathetic with someone's problems can actually make the person feel worse by encouraging them to think negatively about their situation. Instead, it may be inspiring to think of others with disabilities, but who nevertheless have managed to persevere and have good lives (see Chapter 14).

I hesitate to say this, but several times in hospital, particularly when I was in a lot of pain, I did think that it would have been easier if I had died during the operation. This was a totally passive thought, and it was certainly not a wish to die there and then, as I knew that would have made many people very sad. It was more a thought that, if that had happened, then I would be gone, unaware, and no longer suffering all the pain and distress. I think such thoughts should not be taken too seriously as they are fleeting and sporadic, and they are soon gone. All the hospital wards I was in could be very noisy with a lot of moaning and shouting by the patients, and so I would not be surprised if occasional thoughts like that are not uncommon. The thoughts are temporary, and they can be allowed to float away, and be forgotten. Now, much later, when I am feeling a lot better, I am glad simply to be alive. I think of the many things I enjoy and activities that I can do, despite being disabled.

CHAPTER SIX

Vulnerability and hypersensitivity

I REMEMBER THE first time I was lifted out of bed with the electric hoist. I had been lying in bed for a couple of months and was often in pain. When I was lifted into the air for the first time I was very worried the hoist would break and I would go crashing to the floor. Apparently it is not uncommon to worry about this, although the nurses said it was perfectly safe. I think it is natural to feel this kind of fear when the body has been in such a bad state and is alert to any kind of danger.

One day, after I had been in bed in hospital for several months, the physiotherapist suddenly said that we should go outside. I was quite wary and rather doubtful. Once she had wheeled me out and down in the lift to get outside the hospital I was shocked at the cars and ambulances whizzing about, and the frantic activity and movement of people, even though it was a lovely sunny day. It made me feel very nervous after months of lying in bed. It was too much action for my brain to process. But many patients feel shocked when they go outside again into a busy world. I soon said that it was enough and that I was ready to go back up to my bed.

That was not the only time that I have been resistant to change. After many months of being hoisted in and out of bed each day, the staff decided I should use the sliding board and sliding sheet to get from the bed on to the wheelchair and back. I made quite a fuss, fearing that I would fall down on to the floor, and I said, "This feels dangerous, this is torture, why don't we just use the hoist?"

Now, many months later, I am using the sliding board regularly and feel secure and confident. The physiotherapist was right that I just needed to try, and that I would get used to it.

When one is in such a hypersensitive state I think it is best to avoid watching films or reading books that are too demanding or energetic. This is a time to take it gently. For many months in hospital I read only soothing and comforting novels that I had read before, which made me feel much calmer.

I often felt nervous when going outside in the wheelchair or on the electric buggy, especially in the first months after leaving hospital. I felt anxious about bumps on the pavement and crossing the road, worrying that I would fall sideways off the pavement and on to the road. I was on hyper-alert knowing that my body would not be able to react and save me in any emergency. I also could not process images quite normally, and it all seemed very busy and hectic around me. The electric buggy was given to me by Eva's father who is also in a wheelchair. I am now getting used to it and find I am less nervous the more I try. I am even beginning to enjoy the feeling of freedom when I manoeuvre myself about outside on the buggy. It has larger and softer wheels than my wheelchair, and so it is easier to go over bumps on the pavement or road, and it is a smoother ride. I have to steer the buggy myself which is a good mental exercise for me, as I have to be alert and pay attention to all that is going on around me, particularly what is on my left side.

I remember noticing years ago at work that many people thought that they worked harder than the others around them. I thought at the time that they simply could not see how much the others were doing. Everyone can feel how hard they themselves work, but it can be difficult to see what other people manage to get done all day, and also to be aware of what others are feeling, and whether or not they are tired.

I think this may also apply to patients and their carers. The patients are feeling the discomfort and struggle of coping with all the difficulties of the day and are hyper-sensitive to any impatience or implication from others that they could do better. The feeling of total dependence on others puts the patient in a very vulnerable and weak position. Meanwhile, the carers are working hard to solve all the problems. Neither can feel what the other is feeling. They can only observe and try to imagine what the other feels.

It is known that carers can get burnt out by the steady non-stop effort of caring for someone else who cannot look after themselves, and by the responsibility this entails.

It therefore seems important for both the patient and the carer to try to become aware of what the other is going through. People are usually sympathetic with patients, but I think it is also important for patients to try to understand how the carers are feeling. My life has completely changed since my operation in January, and I can see that my husband's life has also changed as a result. He is burdened with having to take over many of the jobs in the house as well as with helping me many times every day. Awareness and acceptance of the struggle we both are going through is important. For the carer it can seem like a never-ending marathon of work, and it can sometimes be exhausting. Although it is hard in a different way, nevertheless the work of the carer is tough, and that needs to be recognised. If the carer can see that you, the patient, are trying as hard as you can, and if you can keep a positive attitude, then that will help him or her feel better and more motivated.

CHAPTER SEVEN

Moving on from trauma

AFTER A FEW months in hospital I suddenly started to feel overwhelmed with a sense of what I had been through earlier in the year. The doctor said that it is not unusual to relive the trauma of the whole experience. I do not have any conscious memory of the first month when I was in intensive care, and so I think this feeling was brought on in part by something more like a body memory. There are nerve cells in many parts of the body, and memories of physical events can be stored in the body as well as in the brain.

I was puzzled at first that I continued with recurrent thoughts about other difficult experiences I have had in my life. I now think that this new trauma of completely losing my independence reawakened something in my brain of memories of old losses. I am glad those feelings have now worn off.

Some people carry traumas within themselves for a very long time, and have what is known as post-traumatic stress disorder. The signs and symptoms as well as the treatments that have been shown to be effective are well described in the book *The Body Keeps the Score* by Bessel Van Der Kolk. The memories of an old physical trauma may be there, while there is little conscious awareness of it. Some patterns get set in the brain, leading to the fear and anxiety that is often seen with post-traumatic stress disorder. The aim is to change those patterns, rewire what was set in the brain and unlearn certain associations. This can be done.

One of the many approaches is treatment with eye movement desensitization and reprocessing (EMDR), which has been shown to be effective in the treatment of post-traumatic stress disorder by helping to change the connections in the brain. Other approaches include neurofeedback, yoga and other physical exercises.

It may help, when going through a bad emotional experience (as opposed to a physical trauma), to feel the feelings in the acute phase with great intensity for a short period of time like 20 minutes, really face the situation and then stop. If this is done a couple of times a day for a few days it can help release the feelings and thus prevent the thoughts from hovering permanently in the back of one's mind and becoming embedded. The aim is eventually to let them go.

The bad pain that I experienced early in 2017 is now over, so I should be able to let the memories go. I certainly do not want to dwell on them. The only gain is to think that, as I feel so very much better than at the beginning of that year, I can expect to continue to improve and have steadily less discomfort.

It can be very difficult to deal with pain, but with the help of painkillers and time, it will become less of a problem. Some other techniques for dealing with pain are discussed in Doidge's book *The Brain That Changes Itself*, and the text on the back cover of the book says: "This will leave you with a sense of wonder at the self-healing power that lies within all of us." This shows us that we can heal in many ways and move on.

CHAPTER EIGHT

Adjusting my expectations and my aims

A FEW MONTHS after coming home, I had a follow-up visit in the hospital and was distressed to hear that 90 percent of the recovery after a spinal cord injury is in the first six months. It was about 10 months since I had had the operation, so that time was up. I was told that my legs are just not strong enough and that 10 percent more improvement will not be enough. I would need five times more strength than I have in order to be able to walk. The doctor said that the possibility of my improving significantly is limited.

Yet again the tears fell down my face. Although it was not the first time I had been told I might not walk again, I suppose that I kept hoping the physiotherapists were wrong. I had been thinking that if I carried on with the exercise bicycle nearly every day for 30 minutes, as I had been doing, then my legs must get stronger. But now I think that perhaps the bicycling leads to a different set of muscles being strengthened, and the muscles in my feet and legs that I really need are just not able to respond.

The spinal cord is not like the brain and it does not recover by itself so easily after an injury. I had heard that the recovery gets slower and slower after a spinal cord injury, but it does keep going.

I had been secretly thinking that, maybe one day. in a couple of years, I might be able to move about, even if not in a very coordinated way. I then realised that it was time for me to begin to face the long-term reality of my probably never walking normally again. I knew that it would be better for me if I could let go of that expectation, and move on, by accepting the situation and focusing instead more on what I can truly expect to be able to do, and how I should go about working towards that. Desperately hoping for something that cannot be is very wearing, so it is best to let that hope fade away and to concentrate on other things. I decided to try to reorient my thoughts to what I may realistically aim for, and think about what I need to work on to reach those goals.

To do more than I can at the moment, then clearly I will need good upper-body strength to lift myself about, while my legs just dangle below me as heavy weights. I am lucky in that my arms are normal and that I can continue working on building the strength in my arms, back and stomach.

I have been told several times that I should focus on whatever I can do to become more independent. I really hope, for example, to be able to get on and off the commode one day by myself, or perhaps on and off the lavatory by myself by using grab rails. Those look like realistic long-term goals that I would be delighted to achieve. Another hope is to get on and off the bed by myself. At least I can get off the exercise bicycle now by myself, and I am working on getting on it by myself. I now realise that I do not need to use all three Velcro straps to attach my feet to the pedals.

I have been told that I could get a special key for public lavatories for the disabled. That would allow me to get out more, and eventually even to go to the cinema, theatre, lectures and concerts (although of course only with help). After over a year spent mostly indoors, the prospect of that sounds amazing.

Everything, I can do by myself, even the little things, helps me feel better, like cutting up vegetables or clearing my breakfast things back into the cupboard and fridge. I also feel very chuffed when I put the kettle on my lap, wheel it along to the sink, fill it up with water, and then manoeuvre in my wheelchair back to the electric base to turn the kettle on to heat, all without spilling a drop of water, or dropping the kettle on the floor.

I can also roll by myself in bed at night from one side to the other, so I can lie for some hours on my left side and then for an hour or so on my right side, which I was told I should do. It is quite a struggle and I do it with some grunting. And when I roll over, my legs just land where they want and are often left rather squashed and twisted. After lying for about an hour on my right side, my right leg often starts to sting, so I just roll back to the other side. This may not sound like much, but it is an achievement for me, which I could not manage some months ago.

I now have what is called a grabber to pick things up off the floor. Several times in hospital I dropped things on to the floor and could not reach down to get them from my wheelchair. I thought such a thing as a grabber must exist, as I knew I would not be the only one with such a problem. There must be many such inventions to help people in wheelchairs. We just need to find them.

When I think back to how I was earlier in 2017 I see how very much better I now feel and am cheered by that, particularly when I think that I may continue to get stronger. I do not feel much pain now, just some stinging in my legs and my feet. It is another world compared with the first few months of 2017, when I needed a lot of painkillers, including morphine. So that is another reason to feel optimistic. I find that as time passes, and the more I can accept the fact of being disabled, the more I can let the old negative memories fade away.

CHAPTER NINE

Letting go of anger, blame and regret

I T IS CRUCIAL not to allow any feelings of resentment, anger or blame take over. It does not help at all to think if only this or that had happened. People sometimes do have bad luck. I saw several patients in hospital who had had accidents that left them in bad shape. There is nothing to be gained from wishing the clock could be turned back to stop the event from having happened. And, even more important, it does not help at all to blame someone else or an organisation, even if they have possibly been negligent or at fault. This will only lead to continuing distress and frustration trying to alter something that has already happened. It cannot be changed. Furthermore, bad feelings of rage and anger in one person will infect others around and leave everyone feeling much worse.

You can choose for yourself how you will react. It is possible to let go of repeated negative thoughts about a situation. You will only end up exhausted and oppressed if they are allowed to hover constantly in the back of your mind. You can move on to a more positive state of mind, and there are various approaches to do this. One is through listening to music, playing a musical instrument or singing. Music therapy is an established intervention which helps people whose lives have been affected by injury, illness or disability. Singing is particularly good as it requires you to breathe in deeply and out again repeatedly, like in yoga, which is also very healing. Light-hearted jokes and seeing comedies may help, as laughing is known be very therapeutic. There are studies showing the benefits of relaxation techniques, such as those mentioned in the book *Doctor You* by Jeremy Howick, and the psychological benefits of being surrounded by nature and enjoying what has been called its "soft fascination".

The overall aim is to develop a good state of mind. It helps to focus on the needs of others and what you can do to help, since compassion (generous feelings of loving kindness) leads to changes in the brain and to greater happiness, more positive emotions, more resilience and a better sense of life purpose.

PART III

EXERCISES, TREATMENTS AND ACTIVITIES

CHAPTER TEN

The importance of exercise

I AM CONVINCED that carrying on doing all of the exercises that have been recommended to me is essential if I want to achieve those goals I can realistically hope to reach. Having grown up in a family in which all of us were very in favour of exercise and sports, it seems natural to take these new exercises very seriously.

When I first arrived at the Oxford Centre for Enablement some patients said that they called the physiotherapy gym the torture chamber. I thought it couldn't be so bad there, as I had always associated exercise with pleasure. However, I now know that many of the exercises are quite tough. It can be very hard work to get those muscles to do anything when there is little or no neurological connection.

I have been trying to do exercises on most days from mid-2017 onwards, but I was told I should do more, particularly to increase my upper body strength. I do my so-called wheelchair yoga, leaning as far down forward as possible for two minutes, and then back up top leaning behind, then out to the right, out to the left, and then twisting around behind me to the right and left. This feels easy as it does not require any leg strength and is using my upper body, which is not damaged. It increases my flexibility and also the strength around my abdomen. I have also been doing daily weightlifting with five different exercises, 20 times with each arm, three times, and I do exercises pulling and stretching using plastic arm bands that work on my back muscles, arms and shoulders. Although my upper body strength is good, I need to work on it a lot more so that I can eventually do more for myself.

It certainly is essential to do a lot of exercises but I think one should watch oneself carefully to avoid overdoing it. I was slowly increasing the weights that I was lifting, starting with 1 kilogram and moving gradually up to 3 kilograms. I then developed a sore shoulder, so I decided it was too much and went back down to 2 kilograms. I recently increased the weights again to 3 kilograms, and then increased them further to 5 kilograms but with fewer repetitions. I hope to increase the weight eventually to 8 kilograms, but again with fewer repetitions, until I am stronger.

We have rented an electric exercise bicycle which is the same as the Motomed machine in the hospital. I do the exercises myself, but the machine tells me how hard I am working, and I can change the resistance level if I want. I always felt that going on the bicycle quite often was doing me good, and that, even if I was developing very little lower leg strength, I was at least strengthening my thighs, and it was giving me some important cardiovascular exercise. Doing as much regular vigorous exercise as possible is very important to stimulate the growth of neurons in the brain and to maintain them. The brain systems require physical movement to generate new cells, so we must keep moving if we can.

We also now have a standing frame at home. I had not realised that it is so important, as I had thought that the exercise bicycle was the main physiotherapy aid that I needed. A standing frame is a tall wooden device that has a base I can stand on and a top wooden surface that I can hold on to tightly to keep my balance. I also have a soft strap to tie me on from behind to stop me from falling. My arms are strong enough that I can pull myself up and balance on the stand. I used to go on the standing frame for about 30 minutes a few times a week while in hospital, and, because it became easy to just balance there and throw an exercise ball back and forth while keeping one hand firmly on the top, I took it for granted. However, after over three months at home without doing any standing, my Achilles tendons shrank considerably, and so when I first got on the frame they I felt very tight, and my blood pressure dropped, making me feel dizzy. I had never known how quickly tendons and ligaments can shrink, and so again I became aware of the importance of keeping going with all the exercises every day if possible. I now go on the standing frame a few times each day for five or ten minutes, and my Achilles tendons have stretched again. We have also discovered that the foot pads on my wheelchair can be adjusted so that the angle between the footpad and the heel is more than the usual 90 degrees. That way my Achilles tendons can be stretched a bit.

I have been told that if I could lose a bit of weight it will be easier for me to lift myself about. Every kilogram less will help. I am not overweight, but I have of course been taking far less exercise than before. I used to go to the gym and to a yoga class once a week, and I usually walked for an hour or more every day with my husband. Plus I went jogging occasionally. I have therefore been making sure in the last months not to eat too much.

I have had foot massage (reflexology) quite a few times and that always feels good. And every evening my carer gives my feet a massage. My feet have been stinging quite a lot for some months, but that seems to be improving. I was told that the massage may help my feet to become desensitised and they will then hurt less. I expect that the massage helps to reawaken normal nerve connections and improve the blood flow. My feet are often very cold, but I hope that the massage will slowly help the blood flow get back to normal.

Some months after coming home, I went to a thermal bath in Bicester and had hydrotherapy for the first time. Floating in the pool was wonderful, with rubber rings around my back and under my arms to support me and prevent me from drowning. Being fully supported by floats can free you, the patient, to make movements which you couldn't otherwise. This can be extremely beneficial, as it helps retrain the body to do certain movements. Swimming, or just moving in water in any way, strengthens you and makes you more flexible, and it is good cardiovascular exercise.

Using the buoyancy and resistance of the water, I could wiggle my hips about, stretch my legs, and move in ways I had not done since the previous January, and I could even pretend I was walking with my feet shovelling slowly along the bottom of the pool. I think it was reminding my brain about doing such movements. It definitely felt beneficial. There is evidence showing that hydrotherapy has positive effects on bones, joints and muscles, and it helps you feel more relaxed.

I have sometimes had small setbacks such as infections and skin problems. This is always rather discouraging as it makes me feel as if I am going backwards. However, it really is a matter of two steps forward and one back. Improvement forwards can start again. For example, I had a pressure sore on my right foot as a result of starting new exercises, and it lasted for some months, making me careful about doing certain exercises and going on the exercise bicycle. The healing was very slow, as the blood flow in my right foot is poor due to my nerve damage, but it eventually healed, just like all the other small problems that I have had. Such slight setbacks are, I think, inevitable and one just has to allow them time to pass.

I also try not to feel too discouraged when I miss a day of exercises or do fewer exercises than usual, as I know I will get back to the usual routine when the various deterrents are gone. I know that all the effort I put into the exercises that I am doing will be very well worth it in the long run.

Activity guidelines for people with a spinal cord injury have been written that describe the types of physical activity that are effective to improve health and fitness, and they provide advice on the frequency, intensity and duration of the physical activity. Details for accessing these guidelines are provided at the end of this book. In addition, lists of physiotherapy exercises that one can do, including in thermal pools, can be downloaded from the organisation Physio Tools online Basic.

It is good to do all the exercises you can with what you've got.

CHAPTER ELEVEN

Getting back to a fairly normal life

QUITE A FEW disabled people are able to get back to work and carry on doing what they love to do, and many do continue to become stronger and more able to manage. Nowadays it is possible to do many things on the computer and telephone without being able to walk.

I remember some years ago asking my niece-in-law, who is an occupational therapist, what this meant she actually did. She said she helped people get back to work. Now, having been with several occupational therapists in the hospital, I understand that it has an even broader scope. I did some painting, woodwork, gardening and photography while there and I enjoyed it, as it felt like normal life. It was opening my mind to doing new things, despite being disabled. The encouragement of the occupational therapists made a big difference and helped me feel more optimistic.

It is possible to start new activities that one has never considered before. For example, I would never have thought I would write a book like this. It had never even remotely crossed my mind that I would ever write a book, but I suddenly started to write several weeks after I came home, and for many months I spent some time every day writing on the computer.

It is also possible nowadays to go out with a wheelchair and to travel to many places in a car or on buses, trains and even aeroplanes. The brochure *Managing Spinal Cord Injury* by the Spinal Injuries Association (SIA) provides valuable information, including guidelines for disabled travellers and how to get an appropriate wheelchair.

I can wheel myself about the house and go to my computer and to the kitchen for meals, and we sometimes go outside if it is warm enough. My four-year-old great-niece asked me how I move my wheelchair, so I demonstrated how I push on the arm rims to go forwards and backwards and how I can go round in a circle. I can wheel myself about well, especially if the floor is smooth and flat and fairly spacious. I sometimes have flashes of awareness of myself as a very different sort of person manoeuvring about the house in my wheelchair. It is peculiar, but I expect that in time it will feel more and more normal.

It is essential to acknowledge and accept the fact of being disabled, and this will also help others to see you dealing with it and coming to terms with the situation. My cousin Jono told me how he once saw a disabled man by the seaside who could only drag himself along the sand, as he couldn't walk. But despite his disability the man managed to play with his small children and they were all laughing and having a very happy time playing together as they rolled about in the sea. The father's disability did not prevent him from having fun with his children and his honesty with himself and therefore with his family was impressive. It is possible for a disabled person to do a lot of fairly normal things with other people, and other people will benefit if they see that the disabled person has a positive and accepting attitude.

CHAPTER TWELVE

Imagining sport and movement

THERE IS RESEARCH showing that just imagining doing a sport can make you better at it and improve your performance. This is based on our ability to know where our body parts are without having to see them. When we visualise ourselves performing a sport, we tap into this sense and teach our bodies to perform better. So when you imagine playing sports, you are actually training your brain in a similar way to what you would when doing the activity.

I have therefore sometimes imagined that I was on a normal bicycle while I was on the exercise bicycle. I also sometimes imagine that I am strolling about while I am on the standing frame. I was told in hospital that I should shift to my right and to my left while on the standing frame to help improve my sense of balance, so I move and wiggle about, and imagine that I am walking normally.

So the question is how imagining movement might apply to physical disabilities. I remembered that I had read about how professional athletes imagine doing their sport and thereby become a lot better at it, and so I googled "imagining sport". Reading on the internet I found that scientists have discovered that just imagining exercising can make you stronger, tone your muscles and delay or stop muscle atrophy. There is a close relationship between imagining and actually doing a movement. The book *The Brain That Changes Itself* has a chapter on imagination which points out that we can change our brain anatomy simply by using our imagination.

Furthermore, it has been shown that it does help to watch the part of the body doing the exercise while simultaneously imagining and thinking about it. The motor regions of the brain thus become stimulated and develop new nerve cells.

It seems that robotic devices might help the brain to understand and relearn some movements by using technology to help patients mimic self-sufficient movements. This may be similar to how I felt in the thermal bath when I could pretend I was walking along the bottom of the pool. Intense focus is required to alter the circuits in the brain and make new connections.

Sometimes, in people with disabilities, the brain switches off the connection with the damaged limb or part of the body that has caused so much pain, and it then ignores it. My new task is to try to increase my awareness of both my legs and both my feet and what they are doing, and to reconnect my mind with my legs and feet.

So, while lying in bed at night, I have been trying to bend my feet up from the toes and then to push them down again, with about 100 movements per foot. I can only manage to bend my feet a few millimetres but it is at least something. Now, having read the publications, I have added in imagining I am moving my feet, and I try to concentrate mentally on the movement. It seems to help, and I feel that I am managing slightly more easily than before. I will certainly persevere with the imagining movements, while simultaneously watching when possible. Neurological studies show that concentrating on the damaged body parts and feeling the subtle connections between the different parts stimulates differentiation between the neurons, which is key to healing.

I now have a new exercise where I go up onto the standing frame and back down on to my wheelchair multiple times. I lift myself with my arms, which do most of the work, but I think simultaneously of pushing on my legs as much as possible, and I try to imagine my legs are participating. I go up and down between five and ten times every day.

I now also see the enormous benefits of having one-to-one help from a physiotherapist who focuses on my particular needs and does specific exercises with me that are suited to my problems, in particular by helping me to practise certain movements with my legs. This is helping me to regenerate some neurological connections, and it helps my muscles relearn, to some extent, how to function.

If there is some small movement in the area that is not functioning properly, like a slight wiggling of the toes, and if you also have feeling in that area, then that is an indication that there is some neurological connection, and this can be built on, leading to some possible further development.

Yoga and meditation exercises often include imagining and visualisation, which lead to greater relaxation and calm, and thus an improvement in health.

It all shows that one can do a lot with the mind to help improve things.

CHAPTER THIRTEEN

Other possible treatments and exercises

We are all aware that going into the bright sunlight makes us feel cheerful, and it seems to do us good. Last summer, on good days, I often went outside to sunbathe, as I felt sure it was helping me generally with healing. The book *The Brain's Way of Healing* has a chapter on rewiring the brain with light. The book mentions the potential benefits of low-level laser treatment (also known as photobiomodulation), a form of light therapy which is often used by professional athletes after an injury. It has been shown to have beneficial effects in the treatment of many different ailments. It works by helping the body marshal its own energy to heal itself, and there are no reported side-effects. There are many scientific studies showing the benefits of low-level laser treatment.

In 2015 I fell over backwards and broke both my wrists trying to avoid a bicyclist. Both my arms were in casts for a couple of months, which led to me getting what is known as a frozen shoulder, an unpleasant disorder which may sometimes last for a year or more. I found a study on the internet where the authors had pooled the data from all the studies on this topic, and they concluded that there were only two effective treatments: injections of cortisone or low-level laser treatment. I then had low-level laser treatment and after a couple of months with about ten sessions it had worked and I was better. Apparently, this treatment has also led to some improvement in animals with spinal cord damage and has been shown to help stroke patients and those with a brain injury

This experience with low-level laser treatment encouraged me. However, I now do not have very high expectations from this therapy, given that my prospects for recovery are not good. Low-level laser therapy helps when the body can do its own natural healing, as it helps speed up the process, but it looks as if my spinal cord injury is not going to heal by itself.

Nevertheless, I think it is worth trying, as I will be pleased by any small improvements, for example if it can help with the hypersensitivity in my right leg which leads to a frequent stinging feeling, or with the poor blood circulation in both feet. See the medical publications in the list of references at the end of this book.

Another topic that is covered in that book is Feldenkrais therapy. This is a form of exercise where one focuses on very tiny and slow body movements while paying careful attention and thinking about what is happening. It is known as awareness through movement. This approach fits with neurological studies showing that concentrating on the damaged body parts stimulates differentiation between the neurons. The slowness of the movement is key for the awareness. I have therefore slowed down and now focus on the movements that I make with my feet every evening while lying in bed. I hope to give my brain a better opportunity to improve the neural connections. I have hardly moved my feet in the last year, and so the area of my brain related to my feet has probably shrunk.

Vitamin B12 has been shown to be beneficial in nerve regeneration, and I now take a daily supplement. Vitamin B12 comes naturally in the animal products that many people eat, including milk products. A good diet is, of course, very important, but I stopped eating any milk products many years ago, and I do not eat much meat. I used to have asthma and required a lot of inhalers. Milk intolerance in adults is not uncommon, and it is sometimes associated with asthma, so I stopped eating any milk products from cows, and I switched to oat milk, rice milk and soya milk. Within a few days I felt better, and since then I have never had any trouble breathing and do not need any inhalers. I have, however, been taking calcium and other supplements to compensate.

It has also been found that omega-3 fatty acids found in natural fish oil help nerve cells communicate better with each other. I have therefore also started taking that supplement, as I want to do all I can to help my nerve cells.

One other topic covered in the book is vision describing the eye exercises developed by William Bates in around 1920. The Bates method is an exercise programme for the eyes designed to strengthen and improve vision. It has received some criticism, but this is probably because it was very ambitious in promising that people could thereby throw away their glasses and see normally without them.

I read about the Bates method many years ago and started to do the exercises regularly, as I am short-sighted and wear glasses. After a few weeks, I saw an optician who told me that the precision of my eyesight was very good and clearly above average. I thought at the time that the exercises had helped me a lot. In recent months I have felt that I cannot see as well as I used to, perhaps because I am not using my eyes in the right way or because my brain damage has led to some inactivity and negligence in looking. I was told in hospital that I should imagine I was a lighthouse and allow my eyes to rove about the room looking at everything, particularly on my left side. The occupational therapist gave me a picture of a lighthouse to put on my bedroom wall to remind me. This was not unlike some of the Bates exercises. Therefore, also inspired by my own earlier experience with the Bates exercises, I now think I will have to add eye exercises to my daily routine.

One other problem that I still have is with my throat. Even after over a year, I still cough a lot and I have a frequent tickling and choking feeling in the back of my throat, and my voice is rather hoarse. I have read that one should try not to cough too much or too violently, as that makes the problem worse. That seems to make sense, so I am trying not to cough and instead drink a lot. I have started gargling with a little warm water with a yogi tea called throat comfort, and I also sometimes let a small liquorice lozenge dissolve slowly in the back of my mouth. The chemicals contained in liquorice are thought to decrease swelling, thin mucus secretions and reduce coughing, and my throat does feel better. I am trying to do what I can to help my throat.

The list of exercises I have is already long, but I am sure I must keep doing them all as much as possible and certainly not slack off.

PART IV

POSTSCRIPT

CHAPTER FOURTEEN

Some admirable people with physical disabilities

I feel encouraged when I think of people I have heard of who have persevered despite their disabilities. Prime examples are of course all the participants in the Paralympics, the Warrior Games and the Invictus Games, who are admirable in how hard they push ahead.

The Paralympics are parallel to the world Olympics, but for people with disabilities. They were created by Ludwig Guttmann, a neurologist at Stoke Mandeville hospital (as shown in the BBC film, *The Best of Men*). The US Warrior Games is a multi-sport event for wounded, injured or ill service personnel and veterans, organised by the US Department of Defense. The Invictus Games is a similar multi-sport event created by the British Prince Harry, in which the participants take part in sports like wheelchair basketball, sitting volleyball and indoor rowing. It is named after the Latin word *invictus*, meaning unconquered or undefeated, which is an excellent name.

I was very impressed by the film *The Miracle Worker* in 1962, about Helen Keller who had an infection when she was 19 months old which left her blind and deaf, and then also dumb. She was a wild little girl who hit and bit people in her frustration at being unable to communicate. A therapist, Anne Sullivan, moved into their house and gradually taught her hand language. She then moved on to speech, practising first by touching water and then showing her how to move her mouth and tongue to create the sounds that matched the concept. Helen Keller later learnt braille and was eventually able to give public talks and became well known. She was the first deaf-blind person to earn a Bachelor of Arts degree in the US, and later she became a political activist and lecturer. She said: "Only through experience of trial and suffering can the soul be strengthened, ambition inspired, and success achieved." "Never bend your head, always hold it high." "Look the world straight in the eye."

Another with great determination is Wolfgang Shaeuble, who was the German finance minister for almost eight years and is now president of the German parliament. He was the target of an assassination attempt at the age of 48 at an election campaign event. His spinal cord was severely injured and he was left paralysed from the attack and has used a wheelchair ever since. Despite this, he has remained an active and very successful politician travelling about in his wheelchair wherever he needs to go. He is a powerful strategic thinker, and is among the most successful politicians in Germany.

Another top politician was Franklin D. Roosevelt, who had polio in 1921 when he was 39 years old and was left permanently paralysed from the waist down. Despite his disability he became president of the US and served as the 32nd president from 1933 until 1945. He founded the National Foundation for Infantile Paralysis, leading to the development of polio vaccines. He said: "Believe you can and you're halfway there." "Keep your eyes on the stars and your feet on the ground." "It is only through labour and painful effort, by grim energy and resolute courage that we move on to better things." "With self-discipline most anything is possible." "Do what you can with what you have, where you are."

Frank Gardner is a well-known British journalist who is currently the BBC's security correspondent.

At the age of 43, while reporting from Saudi Arabia, Gardner was shot and seriously injured in an attack by al-Qaeda sympathisers. Most of the bullets missed his major organs but one hit his spinal cord and he was left partly paralysed in the legs, and since then he has used a wheelchair. Despite his injury he returned to reporting for the BBC, and he continues to work as a reporter, including from abroad. In 2005, he was awarded an OBE for services to journalism and he was voted Person of the Year by the UK *Press Gazette*. He has written three books, and he has resumed skiing using a device that allows disabled people to ski while seated.

Rob Camm was left paralysed from the neck down after a car accident in 2013. The 23-year-old applied for a university place while still in hospital in a spinal unit and he has recently received a first-class honours degree in politics and philosophy. He used voice recognition software to write essays and head movements to control his mouse pointer. He has said: "It's been good to get out of the house and have a purpose." "Many things are possible with some planning." He is now starting a law conversion course at Bristol University.

Matthew Hampson became a tetraplegic (having paralysis of all four limbs and torso) at the age of 20 after a rugby practice accident while playing for the England under-21 rugby team. He now requires a ventilator to breathe. He divides his time between raising money for spinal care both for himself and others, including the UK charity Spinal Research. He aims to inspire and support young people seriously injured through sport, and he regularly visits beneficiaries, schools and societies where he gives advice and motivational talks based on his own experiences.

Anne Dreydel was badly injured at the age of 22 when a bomb fell on her London home during the second world war. The explosion paralysed her from the waist down, and she remained in a wheelchair for the rest of her life. She studied English at St Anne's College in Oxford and then German in Bonn during her holidays. In 1947 she co-founded the Oxford-Bonn Universities Committee to develop the twinning of Oxford and Bonn, which encouraged students from Germany to study in Oxford. She co-founded the Oxford English Centre, which became St Clare's College in Oxford, and she was the principal. She also later became the head of the American International School of Florence and then the director of the Oxford Centre for Learning Skills. She helped disabled people by serving on the Committee for the Employment of Disabled People for Oxfordshire and Berkshire. She was awarded the German Federal Cross of Merit (Bundesverdienstkreuz), and was awarded an OBE for her services to education.

Stephen Hawking, was a well-known theoretical physicist and cosmologist. He had a rare early-onset slow-progressing form of motor neurone disease, diagnosed when he was 21. It gradually paralysed him over the decades, but, despite this, he continued to work, and he had an extremely impressive record. He was a recipient of the Presidential Medal of Freedom, the highest civilian award in the US. In 2002 he was ranked 25th in the BBC's poll of the 100 greatest Britons. He also achieved commercial success with his works of popular science. He communicated using a single cheek muscle attached to a speech-generating device. In 2007 he took part in a zero-gravity flight, in part he said, "to show that people need not be limited by physical handicaps as long as they are not disabled in spirit". And he said: "However difficult life may seem, there is always something you can do and succeed at".

All of the above people provide amazing examples of determination, and they show us that we need not be prevented from doing much of what we love to do, even if we are disabled. People have very different interests and very different problems, but there is much that can be done, and we should all aim to follow the paths that really interest us. Disabilities may prevent us from doing some things, but the possibilities are there to pursue fascinating projects, particularly given new technology and some clever inventions to help us. Modern technology provides a wide range of options for people with disabilities, and there are many examples of people who have benefited.

CHAPTER FIFTEEN

*A brief history of my life before the operation,
with some factors helping me to develop a positive
attitude in the face of obstacles*

I am adding this, as you, the reader, may like to know a bit about who I am and what my background is. I was born in Australia in 1950, and shortly thereafter we returned to England before going to Uganda for two years. This was followed by another sea journey back to Australia. We spent the next eight years in Canberra and I have many good memories of picnics by the river, holidays at the seaside, and of course the usual Australian encouragement to be tough and sort things out for yourself. My two brothers and I were taught for example to be very careful about snakes, spiders and sharks, and were told that if we ever got lost, we should stay where we were, and sing all the songs we remember and then sing them all over again. This is to help the parents find the lost child and to stop them wandering even further away.

Some children do wander off and get lost every year in the Australian outback. Our first house was on the edge of Canberra and across the road there was simply wild space, extending for miles, so we could just roam about at leisure and play. At the time Canberra was like a small country town and was many miles from almost anywhere.

Winters we skied in the Snowy Mountains, and every summer we went to Wimby Beach near Batemans Bay, where we stayed in a little house with no electricity. The area was very deserted, with hardly anyone about except us. We used to go fishing from the beach with all five of us in a tiny rowing boat. We did exciting things like put out a large barrel on the sea with an anchor attached and fish heads on a large hook to catch sharks off the beach where we used to swim. We (meaning my father and a family friend) caught a bronze whaler shark, which was about 4–5 feet long, a baby great white shark which was about 7 feet long, and finally a grey nurse shark, which was about 4–5 feet long. The baby great white shark had been half eaten by other sharks and was dead, but I remember that as our family friend was pulling it up, he gave a shriek and let it drop. We could see the large shark's head a couple of feet below us, as if it were looking right at us. They then quickly rowed us children back to the beach in the little rowing boat, so we were safe.

My parents said the shark was delicious. Not many people have eaten a great white shark. Usually it is the other way around.

My father then had sabbatical leave from the university and we travelled briefly to Hong Kong, where my mother had spent her childhood, then England, and then Cold Spring Harbor on Long Island, New York, for six months, before going back to Australia.

My sense of direction has always been poor and I am often not very aware of what is around me, so moving country so often in my life did sometimes leave me feeling anxious and worried about getting lost and left behind, especially when I was young. The one number that is still most firmly stored in my brain is the telephone number of our house in Canberra, which shows how worried I was.

We later moved back to Cold Spring Harbor, where we spent the next ten years. We lived in a house just above a beach off the Long Island Sound. This came with my father's position as director of the Cold Spring Harbor laboratory. My brothers and I went to the local school, had summer jobs in the lab and absorbed much of the American belief that you can set your own goals and get things done if you put the effort into it. I then went to Smith College in Massachusetts, where my mother encouraged me to major in mathematics, as I liked it and she thought it would be useful. Her mother had been an active feminist and fought for women's rights most of her adult life, often in the face of some resistance. Smith College is an all-women's college that supports women in becoming independent. Both my brothers went to Brown University and later studied medicine, so are now doctors.

We moved back to England and I went to the London School of Economics and Political Science (LSE), where I studied statistics. I got my MSc and PhD and moved on to various jobs as a medical statistician. My husband and I met at the LSE, and we moved together to Munich and then Florida, and later Kronberg in Germany where he had grown up.

Unfortunately I could not have any children, but I have four lovely godchildren, three nephews and a niece. Of course I minded a lot not being able to have children. I decided that as there was nothing I could do about it, I would really make an effort not to dwell on it too much. I try to think that if nothing can be done about a bad situation, then it is best to try not to allow the distressing thoughts to dominate.

I very much enjoyed working for the Germany pharmaceutical company Hoechst AG in Frankfurt, which after various mergers became Aventis and then Sanofi.

First, I was project statistician in cardiovascular drug development and worked on ramipril (a drug which I took for many months in 2007 for my heart). This involved the design of clinical trials, the statistical analysis of the results, writing up the study reports on the efficacy and safety of the drugs, and helping to prepare summary documents for the health authorities which would decide whether the drugs would be approved. I then became head of the Frankfurt group of statisticians and later head of the Frankfurt department of Biostatistics, Data Management and Statistical Programming.

In 1998 I caught Lyme disease from a tick in our garden. It was a few months before I received effective antibiotic treatment, so I developed what is known as post-treatment Lyme disease syndrome, and I remained ill for nearly five years. I had been told I would eventually get better and so I was patient, although it was a shock when I heard that it might take three years or more. This was my first real exercise in developing the right mental attitude towards dealing with a long-term physical problem. I did remain fairly cheerful throughout that time, and tried to use the time productively, for example by writing a paper on Lyme disease. I knew that post-treatment Lyme disease syndrome was a hotly debated and quite controversial topic at that time, so I decided to look into the published literature on it, and explore what I could. I had worked for over 20 years in medical statistics, so it was a familiar enterprise. I collected all the relevant medical publications and pooled the data to produce a complete summary of the information. This was what is known as a meta-analysis, and the paper was later published.

When it became clear that I was still too ill to continue in my old position, I agreed to leave the company. Sometime later, when I was stronger, I was able to start working freelance part-time from home as a statistical consultant for the German pharmaceutical company Boehringer Ingelheim, and also for an epidemiology institute run by a friend.

I may have had residual heart damage, as Lyme disease can sometimes affect the heart. I first started noticing having irregular heartbeats in 2001 and then continued to have palpitations intermittently for some years. It is possible that Lyme disease was the cause of my atrial fibrillation, for which I had the operation that went so badly wrong. At least my heart rhythm now seems to be normal again after the operation.

In 2015 (as mentioned above) I fell over backwards trying to avoid a bicyclist who was racing across a bridge towards me, and I broke both my wrists. With both arms in casts I then had my first adult experience of depending totally on others for help. I did all the recommended exercises for my wrists, and after a couple of months I had recovered enough to manage to do most things again by myself.

I have had some difficulties in my life, but I have also have had many very good times, and have had quite a lot of good luck. I had an interesting upbringing, as well as a good education and fulfilling jobs. My husband and I now live in England.

CHAPTER SIXTEEN

Writing this book

Writing this book has felt like a great cathartic release for me, and it has helped me to focus on key topics. Sometime after I came home from hospital, the idea of writing a book started hovering in the back of my mind. Several weeks later, on the day after I had dreamt I stood and took three little steps shuffling forward, I realised what my first sentence would be, and I sat at my computer and wrote Chapter 1. I continued to think about it regularly over the next months. The book has surged out, and it feels like I have now dealt with the ordeal of last year. Perhaps this was what my brain needed to do in order to process what I have been through, and to settle it all quietly away. Much of what I have written seems to have been thought up without my conscious control. Apparently, there are millions of processes going on in the brain at any one time, but we are unconscious of much of what the brain does.

I remember once in college, when I had a difficult mathematical theorem to prove, I sat for about an hour or more on the homework trying out different approaches, but without success. I then went swimming in a lake with a friend. Several hours later, not having being aware that I had been thinking about the mathematics at all, I came back to my room, sat at my desk and just wrote out the solution. It seems that part of my brain had been working on the problem while we were out, and it had found the solution without me being aware of it. Those mathematical abilities I once had are now gone, but I do realise that my brain does sometimes quietly sort out some problems without me noticing it doing any work. It seems as if the brain first has to be primed and given a task. It then needs the space and freedom to sort things out. Of course one has to put the energy into it, but the brain then seems to get to work. It is like when one cannot remember a name or a word. It is stored in there somewhere, and after waiting a little while it suddenly comes back.

Now that the right side of my brain is a bit damaged and not functioning as well as before, I have become more aware of differences between parts of my brain.

Years ago when I was working, sometimes part of my brain would suddenly remind me in the middle of the night about something I needed to do, and then what felt like a more conscientious part of my brain remembered in the morning and made sure the task was done. It also happened recently when my brain told me in the middle of the night that I had not taken my blood-thinning medication the day before, so I took it the next day.

I have been aware that part of my brain was busily thinking up phrases for this book every night over the last months, and that what felt like a different part of my brain was noticing, remembering and ready to write it out in the morning.

The book is now finished, and it has been released. One day soon I hope to start new projects, think about other things and move on. The options are open.

APPENDIX

REFERENCES

ORGANISATIONS
PROVIDING SUPPORT
AND ADVICE

DISABILITY
EQUIPMENT

REFERENCES

Books

Doidge, Norman. 2008. *The Brain That Changes Itself*. London: Penguin Books.

Doidge, Norman. 2015. *The Brain's Way of Healing*. London: Penguin Random House.

Howick, Jeremy. 2017. *Doctor You: Introducing the Hard Science of Self-healing*. London: Hodder and Stoughton.

Thondup, Tulku. 1998. *The Healing Power of Mind*. Boston, MA, and London: Shambhala Publications.
Van der Kolk, Bessel. 2014. *The Body Keeps the Score: Mind, Brain and Body in the Transformation of Trauma*. London: Penguin Books.

Medical publications

Note: These medical publications can be found by searching "PubMed" on the internet (Link: https://www.ncbi.nlm.nih.gov/pubmed), and entering, for example, the surname of the first author with the initial of the first name and perhaps a key word, or by entering the title of the article. The abstracts summarising the main points are usually available, and the full publication can sometimes be downloaded free, or bought.

Treatment for post-traumatic stress disorder

Chen Y-R, Hung K-W, Tsai J-C, et al. Efficacy of Eye-Movement Desensitization and Reprocessing for Patients with Posttraumatic-Stress Disorder: A Meta-Analysis of Randomized Controlled Trials. Chao L, ed. *PLoS ONE*. 2014;9(8):e103676. doi:10.1371/journal.pone.0103676.

Gallegos AM, Crean HF, Pegeon WE, Heffner, KL. Meditation and yoga for posttraumatic stress disorder: A meta-analytic review of randomized controlled trials. *Clin Psychol Rev* 2017 Dec;58:115-124. doi:10.1016/j.cpr.2017.10.004.

Van der Kolk BA, Hodgdon H, Gapen M, Musicaro R, Suvak MK, Hamlin E, et al. (2016) Randomized Controlled Study of Neurofeedback for Chronic PTSD. *PLoS ONE*. 2016. 11(12): e0166752. doi:10.1371/journal.pone.0166752.

Imagining sport and movement

Di Rienzo F, Debarnot U, Daligault S, et al. Online and Offline Performance Gains Following Motor Imagery Practice: A

Comprehensive Review of Behavioral and Neuroimaging Studies. *Frontiers in Human Neuroscience*. 2016;10:315. doi:10.3389/fnhum.2016.00315.

Holanda LJ, Silva PMM, Amorim TC, Lacerda MO, Simão CR, Morya E. Robotic assisted gait as a tool for rehabilitation of individuals with spinal cord injury: a systematic review. *Journal of NeuroEngineering and Rehabilitation*. 2017;14:126. doi:10.1186/s12984-017-0338-7.

Slimani M, Tod D, Chaabene H, Miarka B, Chamari K. Effects of Mental Imagery on Muscular Strength in Healthy and Patient Participants: A Systematic Review. *Journal of Sports Science & Medicine*. 2016;15(3):434-450.

Wright DJ, McCormick SA, Williams J, Holmes PS. Viewing Instructions Accompanying Action Observation Modulate Corticospinal Excitability. *Frontiers in Human Neuroscience*. 2016;10:17. doi:10.3389/fnhum.2016.00017.

Exercises for people with a spinal cord injury
Van der Scheer JW, Martin Ginis KA, Ditor DS, Goosey-Tolfrey VL, Hicks AL, West CR, Wolfe DL. Effects of exercise on fitness and health of adults with spinal cord injury: A systematic review. *Neurology*. 2017;89:736-745.
Link: http://www.ncsem-em.org.uk/wp-content/uploads/2017/10/Spinal-cord-injury-guidelines.pdf

Thermal baths

Mooventhan A, Nivethitha L. Scientific Evidence-Based Effects of Hydrotherapy on Various Systems of the Body. *North American*

Journal of Medical Sciences. 2014;6(5):199-209. doi:10.4103/1947-2714.132935.

The benefits of music, laughter, nature and compassion

Altenmüller E, Schlaug G. Apollo's gift: new aspects of neurologic music therapy. *Progress in brain research*. 2015;217:237-252. doi:10.1016/bs.pbr.2014.11.029.

Berk LS, Tan SA, Fry WF, Napier BJ, Lee JW, Hubbard RW, Lewis JE, Ebt WC. Neuroendocrine and stress hormone changes during mirthful laughter. *Am J Med Sci* 1989 Dec;298(6):390-6. Joye Y, Pals R, Steg L, Evans BL New Methods for Assessing the Fascinating Nature of Nature Experiences. *PLoS ONE* 2013. 8(7): e65332. https://doi.org/10.1371/journal.pone.0065332.

Fredrickson BL, Cohn MA, Coffey KA, Pek J, Finkel SM. Open hearts build lives: positive emotions, induced through loving-kindness meditation, build consequential personal resources. J *Pers Soc Psychol*. 2008 Nov;95(5):1045-1062. doi:10.1037/a0013262.

Low-level laser treatment

Chung H, Dai T, Sharma SK, Huang Y-Y, Carroll JD, Hamblin MR. The Nuts and Bolts of Low-level Laser (Light) Therapy. *Annals of Biomedical Engineering*. 2012;40(2):516-533. doi:10.1007/s10439-011-0454-7.

Hashmi JT, Huang Y-Y, Osmani BZ, Sharma SK, Naeser MA, Hamblin MR. Role of Low-Level Laser Therapy in Neurorehabilitation. *PM & R: the journal of injury, function, and rehabilitation.* 2010;2(12 Suppl 2):S292-S305. doi:10.1016/j.pmrj.2010.10.013.

Salehpour F, Mahmoudi J, Kamari F, et al. Brain Photobiomodulation Therapy: A Narrative Review. *Mol Neurobiol* (2018). https://doi.org/10.1007/s12035-017-0852-4.

Vitamin B12 for nerve regeneration

Gröber U, Kisters K, Schmidt J. Neuroenhancement with Vitamin B12 – Underestimated Neurological Significance. *Nutrients.* 2013;5(12):5031-5045. doi:10.3390/nu5125031.

Sun H, Yang T, Li Q, et al. Dexamethasone and vitamin B_{12} synergistically promote peripheral nerve regeneration in rats by upregulating the expression of brain-derived neurotrophic factor. *Archives of Medical Science : AMS.* 2012;8(5):924-930. doi:10.5114/aoms.2012.31623.

The benefits of Omega-3 fish oil

Fiala M, Halder RC, Sagong B, Ross O, Sayre J, Porter V, Bredesen DE. ω-3 Supplementation increases amyloid-β phagocytosis and resolvin D1 in patients with minor cognitive impairment. *FASEB J* 2015 Jul;29(7):2681-9. doi: 10.1096/fj.14-264218. Epub 2015 Mar 24.

Jeromson S, Gallagher IJ, Galloway SDR, Hamilton DL. Omega-3 Fatty Acids and Skeletal Muscle Health. Smith V, ed. *Marine Drugs.* 2015;13(11):6977-7004. doi:10.3390/md13116977.

Molfino A, Gioia G, Fanelli FR, Muscaritoli M. The Role for Dietary Omega-3 Fatty Acids Supplementation in Older Adults. *Nutrients.* 2014;6(10):4058-4072. doi:10.3390/nu6104058.

u H, Guo Y, Zhang W, et al. Omega-3 polyunsaturated fatty acid supplementation improves neurologic recovery and attenuates white matter injury after experimental traumatic brain injury. *Journal of Cerebral Blood Flow & Metabolism*. 2013;33(9):1474-1484. doi:10.1038/jcbfm.2013.108.

Sources for quotations in chapters 3, 9 and 14

Camm, Rob:
https://www.bbc.co.uk/news/uk-england-40605793

Hawking, Stephen:
https://www.brainyquote.com/quotes/stephen_hawking_627103
https://www.nytimes.com/2018/03/14/world/europe/stephen-hawking-quotes.html

Keller, Helen:
https://www.brainyquote.com/lists/authors/top_10_helen_keller_quotes.

Roosevelt, Franklin D.:
https://www.brainyquote.com/authors/theodore_roosevelt

Soft fascination of nature:
https://en.wikipedia.org/wiki/Attention_restoration_theory

Star Trek and **Superman** quotations are from the films *Star Trek* and *Superman* in the 1960s.

ORGANISATIONS PROVIDING SUPPORT AND ADVICE

Note: Most of these organisations are in the UK, but there will be similar organisations in other countries.

Age UK is the UK's largest charity working with older people. Link: www.ageuk.org.uk. Telephone: 0800 055 6112.

Back Up is a charity that delivers a range of services to build confidence and independence back into the lives of people with a spinal cord injury. They provide, among other things, courses in wheelchair use to improve the skills of the disabled person. Link: https://www.backuptrust.org.uk. Telephone: 020 8875 1805.

Brain Injury Rehabilitation Trust (BIRT) is a charity which aims to provide the best quality neurobehavioural rehabilitation for people with complex and challenging needs after a brain injury. Link: https://www.thedtgroup.org/brain-injury.

Care UK is the UK's largest independent provider of health and social care. Link: http://www.careuk.com. Telephone: 03702 185 407.

Enrych is an organisation that is looking beyond disability. It supports adults with a disability to live the most active and independent lives possible. It does this through leisure, learning and sporting activities with Enrych volunteers, and it also offers a personal assistant service in some areas. Link: https://enrych. org.uk. Telephone: 01926 485446.

International Spinal Cord Society is a non-profit organisation, whose purpose is to study all problems relating to lesions of the spinal cord. It was founded by Ludwig Guttmann, who created the Paralympics. Link: .

PhysioTools Online Basic provides lists of different physiotherapy exercises, and the lists can usually be downloaded by registered physiotherapists to create a personalised exercise programme. Link: .

Spinal Injuries Association (SIA) is a national user-led spinal cord injuries charity. Link: www.spinal.co.uk/about-us. Telephone: 0800 980 0501. The SIA has written the helpful brochure *Managing Spinal Cord Injury: Continuing Care*, which can be bought directly from it. Link: https://www.spinal.co.uk/ product/managing-spinal-cord-injury-continuing-care. It also has an online learning tool to help members better understand the complexities of making a successful NHS continuing healthcare application.

Wheel Power is a charity that provides opportunities for disabled people to get into sport and lead active lives. Link: .

DISABILITY EQUIPMENT

Valuable information on disability equipment is available from the Disabled Living Foundation. Link: www.dlf.org.uk. See their list of fact sheets.

Note: Some of the following gadgets and devices are available from organisations in the UK, but there will be similar organisations that provide them in other countries.

Bed levers that can be used to replace the normal hospital bed rails. They provide a similar barrier and support to use when manoeuvring about on the bed, but they only extend a short distance, allowing space for the patient to get out of bed. (They can be obtained from the NHS, or bought via Amazon).

Bedside bell, electric, to ring in another room in the house. It can be bought via Amazon.

Cushion, "Repose". It is air-inflated, and could be used for outdoor use on a wheelchair or an electric buggy to buffer the effects of the bumps on the pavement. It is available from the NHS, or it can be bought via Amazon.

Exercise bicycle, electric, "MotoMed Viva2", which can be rented or bought from MediMotion Ltd. Link: www.motomed. com. Telephone: 01559 384097.

Grab rails to attach to a wall for secure lifting using arm strength.

Grabber to pick items up from the floor. It can be bought via Amazon.

Key to the UK public lavatories for the disabled. This can be obtained from the local UK council.

Lavatory, features that may be put on the lavatory that may enable a transfer directly from the wheelchair, using grab rails.

Leg lifter, to hook one end around a foot and then pull the leg up and move it using the arms. It may be provided by the NHS, or it can be bought via Amazon.

Parking badge, disabled, that makes it easier to find a suitable parking space when out in the car. It can be obtained from the local UK council.

Personal alarm to wear around the neck, for emergencies, to call a local organisation that has a front door key. It can be obtained via the organisation Age UK.

Shoes: Ugg boots, made by Ugg, have a soft sheepskin lining and solid non-slip sole. Warm and good for winter use and to prevent pressure sores. **Skechers** is a company making shoes with a soft lining and solid non-slip sole. They are lighter and good for summer use.

Sliding sheet and banana board to move from the wheelchair to the commode and back and from the chair to the bed and back. They are provided by the NHS, or can be bought via Amazon.

Sockaid that can be used to help put on compression socks. It can be obtained from the NHS, or bought via Amazon).

Standing frame, wooden, which can be bought from the company Oswestry in Wrexham, North Wales. Link: http://www.oswestry-frames.co.uk. Telephone: 01691 718218.

Video door entry kit to see visitors, speak to them and then open the front door. It can be bought via Amazon.

Weights to practise weight-lifting using the arms. Different-sized weights can be bought via Amazon.

Wheelchair, standard, which is provided by the NHS. Other wheelchairs specifically for people with a spinal cord injury can be bought which may be lighter, narrower, and possibly with a simpler footpad which is less cumbersome. The Spinal Injuries Association has centres where one can try out different types of wheelchair.

Abbreviations
BIRT: Brain Injury Rehabilitation Trust
NHS: National Health Service
SIA: Spinal Injuries Association
UK: United Kingdom
US: United States